Low Cholesterol Recipes

Delicious Food Options to Keep Cholesterol in Check

BY: SOPHIA FREEMAN

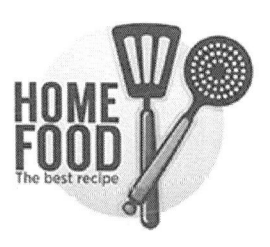

© 2019 Sophia Freeman All Rights Reserved

COPYRIGHTED

Liability

This publication is meant as an informational tool. The individual purchaser accepts all liability if damages occur because of following the directions or guidelines set out in this publication. The Author bears no responsibility for reparations caused by the misuse or misinterpretation of the content.

Copyright

The content of this publication is solely for entertainment purposes and is meant to be purchased by one individual. Permission is not given to any individual who copies, sells or distributes parts or the whole of this publication unless it is explicitly given by the Author in writing.

* * * * * ★ ★ ★ ★ ★ * *

My gift to you!

Thank you, cherished reader, for purchasing my book and taking the time to read it. As a special reward for your decision, I would like to offer a gift of free and discounted books directly to your inbox. All you need to do is fill in the box below with your email address and name to start getting amazing offers in the comfort of your own home. You will never miss an offer because a reminder will be sent to you. Never miss a deal and get great deals without having to leave the house! Subscribe now and start saving!

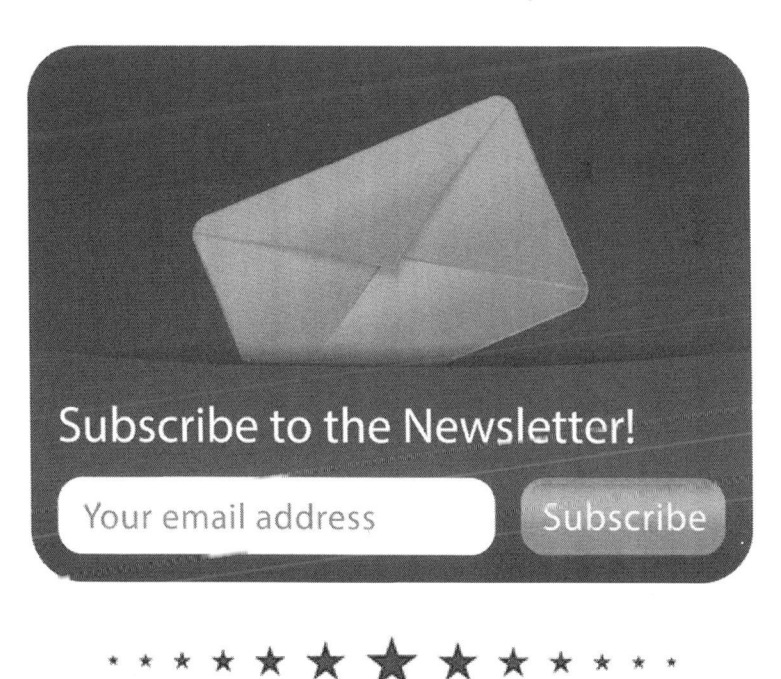

Table of Contents

Chapter I: Low Cholesterol Poultry and Meat Recipes 7

    1) Slow Cooker Pulled Pork 8

    2) Mongolian Beef and Spring Onions................................. 9

    3) Penne with Chicken and Asparagus.............................. 12

    4) Doreen's Ham Slices on the Grill 15

    5) Turkey Veggie Meatloaf Cups 17

Chapter II: Low Cholesterol Seafood Recipes........................ 19

    6) Cod with Italian Crumb Topping.................................. 20

    7) Mustard Tuna Salad 22

    8) Garlic Basil Shrimp.. 24

    9) Grilled Cilantro Salmon 26

    10) Parmesan Crusted Tilapia 28

Chapter III: Low Cholesterol Beverages and Snacks 30

    11) Summer Breeze.. 31

12) Baked Sweet Potato Fries 32

13) Peach Medley 34

14) Crunchy Onion Rings 36

15) Viva Forever! 38

Chapter IV: Low Cholesterol Vegetarian Recipes 40

16) Roasted Harvest Vegetables 41

17) French Ratatouille 44

18) Balsamic and Olive Oil Roasted Brussels sprouts 46

19) Creamy Corn Casserole 48

20) All-Vegetable Soup 50

Chapter V: Low Cholesterol Desserts................................... 53

21) Mango Raspberry Sorbet 54

22) Chocolate Chip Oatmeal Cookies 56

23) Pumpkin Mousse 59

24) Zesty Lemon Bars 60

25) Strawberry Fluff 62

About the Author 64

Author's Afterthoughts 66

Chapter I: Low Cholesterol Poultry and Meat Recipes

zzzzzzzzzzzzzzzzzzzzzzzzzzzzzzzzzzzzzzzzzz

1) Slow Cooker Pulled Pork

This delicious recipe is one to fall in love with. The recipe has only 49 mg of cholesterol. The pork simmered in root beer gives it a unique flavor.

Preparation Time: 7 hours and 10 minutes

Makes: 8 servings

Ingredient List:

- 1 pork tenderloin (2 pounds)
- 1 bottle of your favorite barbecue sauce (18 ounces)
- 1 bottle or can root beer (12 fluid ounces)
- 8 hamburger buns (split and toast them lightly)

zzzzzzzzzzzzzzzzzzzzzzzzzzzzzzzzzzzzzzzzzzzz

Instructions:

Take a slow cooker and put the pork tenderloin in it. Pour the root beer on it and let the meat cook on the low heat for 6 to 7 hours until the pork can be shredded easily. After that, drain the pork well. Pour barbecue sauce over it and serve with hamburger buns.

2) Mongolian Beef and Spring Onions

This beautiful recipe is perfect for people who love beef and rice. It's the perfect combination of both with just 27 mg of cholesterol. Just follow the recipe and eat this yummy dish with boiled or fried rice.

Preparation Time: 30 minutes

Makes: 4 servings

Ingredient List:

- Beef flank steak (1 pound) (slice it ¼-inch-thick on the diagonal)
- Vegetable oil (1 cup plus 2 teaspoons)
- Grated fresh ginger root (½ teaspoons)
- Green onions (2 bunches) (cut them in 2 inches in length)
- Finely chopped garlic (1 tablespoon)
- Cornstarch (¼ cup)
- Soy sauce (½ cup)
- Water (½ cup)
- Dark brown sugar (2/3 cup)

zzzzzzzzzzzzzzzzzzzzzzzzzzzzzzzzzzzzzzzzzz

Instructions:

Take a saucepan and heat 2 teaspoons of vegetable in it over medium heat. Stir in ginger and garlic until they leave a scent. Add water, brown sugar and soy sauce. Increase the heat and stir the mixture for 4 minutes. When the sugar dissolves and the sauce thickens, remove it from heat and put it aside.

Take a bowl and add beef into it. Stir in cornstarch. Leave the meat for 10 minutes for the cornstarch to absorb all the juice of the meat. Heat oil in a deep-sided skillet. Shake off the excess cornstarch from the beef slices and then drop them in the oil. Fry the slices for 2 minutes until the edges start to brown. Collect the beef slices on paper towels for the oil to dry. Remove the oil from the skillet and return it to the stove over medium heat. Stir in the beef slices again over medium heat. Add the sauce to the beef slices and stir to combine.

3) Penne with Chicken and Asparagus

This recipe is perfect for pasta and chicken lovers. This recipe contains only 20 mg of cholesterol. I promise you would want to eat this dish every day.

Preparation Time: 35 minutes

Makes: 8 servings

Ingredient List:

- 2 skinless, boneless chicken breast halves (cut them into cubes)
- 1 package dried penne pasta (16 ounces)
- Garlic powder (to taste)
- Divided olive oil (5 tablespoons)
- Salt
- Pepper
- Low-sodium chicken broth (½ cup)
- Slender asparagus spears (1 bunch) (trim them and then cut them on diagonal into 1-inch pieces)
- 1 thinly sliced garlic clove
- Parmesan cheese (¼ cup)

zzzzzzzzzzzzzzzzzzzzzzzzzzzzzzzzzzzzzzzzzzz

Instructions:

Lightly salt a large pot of water and bring it to boil. Cook the pasta in the boiled water for 10 minutes. Drain the pasta and set it aside. Over medium-high heat, heat 3 tablespoons of olive oil. Add chicken and sprinkle garlic powder, salt and pepper over it. Stir and cook the chicken until it's thoroughly cooked and browned.

Collect the chicken on paper towels. Pour the chicken broth into the same skillet and add garlic, asparagus, a pinch of garlic powder, pepper and salt. Cover the skillet and let the broth cook for 10 minutes until the asparagus is soft.

Add the chicken to the broth. Stir. Now add this chicken mixture to the pasta and mix well. Let the mixture sit for 5 minutes and drizzle over it 2 tablespoons of olive oil. Garnish with Parmesan cheese!

4) Doreen's Ham Slices on the Grill

With only 8 mg of cholesterol, this recipe is an all-time favorite of my family. I sometimes replace it with turkey slices too and it's absolutely heavenly.

Preparation Time: 25 minutes

Makes: 4 servings

Ingredient List:

- 2 slices ham
- Packed brown sugar (1 cup)
- Prepared horseradish (1/3 cup)
- Lemon juice (¼ cup)

zzzzzzzzzzzzzzzzzzzzzzzzzzzzzzzzzzzzzzzzzzzzz

Instructions:

Heat your outdoor grill over high heat. Oil the grate lightly. Mix lemon juice, brown sugar and prepared horseradish in a small bowl. Heat this mixture in a microwave oven for 1 minute until it is warm. Score the ham slices and place the slices on the grill.

Pour the mixture from the oven over the ham slices while they grill. Grill each side of the slices for 8 minutes. Serve when they are cooked through. Enjoy!

5) Turkey Veggie Meatloaf Cups

If you are a turkey fan, this recipe would make your day. With only 47 mg of cholesterol, this dish would be your next love. I, personally, never get enough of this yummy recipe.

Preparation Time: 50 minutes

Makes: 10 servings

Ingredient List:

- Extra lean ground turkey (1 pound)
- Roughly chopped zucchini (2 cups)
- 1 roughly chopped red bell pepper
- Roughly chopped onions (1 ½ cups)
- Uncooked couscous (½ cup)
- Dijon mustard (1 tablespoon)
- Worcestershire sauce (2 tablespoons)
- Barbecue sauce (½ cup)
- 1 egg
- Cooking spray

zzzzzzzzzzzzzzzzzzzzzzzzzzzzzzzzzzzzzzzzzzzz

Instructions:

Set the oven to 400F. Apply cooking spray on 20 muffin cups. Blend zucchini, red bell pepper and onions in a food processor until they are finely chopped. Don't puree them. Take a bowl and mix vegetables, ground turkey, egg, Worcestershire sauce, Dijon mustard and couscous.

Add this mixture in the muffin cups. Fill them to the 3/4th. Spread barbecue sauce on each cup. Bake them in the oven for 25 minutes. Check the internal temperature of the muffins. It should be 160F. Before you serve the muffins, let them sit for 5 minutes.

Chapter II: Low Cholesterol Seafood Recipes

zzzzzzzzzzzzzzzzzzzzzzzzzzzzzzzzzzzzzzzzzzzz

6) Cod with Italian Crumb Topping

Absolutely delicious!!! This is a quick cod recipe that has low fat and only 39 mg of cholesterol. If you want to keep your cholesterol level to the minimum and enjoy seafood, this recipe would serve that purpose.

Preparation Time: 25 minutes

Makes: 4 servings

Ingredient List:

- 4 cod fillets (3 ounces each)
- Cornmeal (1 tablespoon)
- Grated Parmesan cheese (2 tablespoons)
- Fine dry bread crumbs (¼ cup)
- Olive oil (1 teaspoon)
- Garlic powder (1/8 teaspoons)
- Ground black pepper (1/8 teaspoons)
- Italian seasoning (½ teaspoons)
- 1 lightly beaten egg white
- Cooking spray

zz

Instructions:

First of all, set your oven at 450F. Now, take a small bowl and mix breadcrumbs, cornmeal, cheese, oil, garlic powder, pepper and Italian seasoning. Set aside. Grease the broiling rack of your broiler.

Put the cod on the rack. Brush it with the egg white and evenly spread the crumbs mixture on it. Now bake the fish fillets in the oven for 12 minutes. Check with a fork if it's opaque throughout. Enjoy!

7) Mustard Tuna Salad

This absolutely delicious recipe contains just 25 mg of cholesterol. You would love the combination of tuna with different kinds of mustard. This salad is light and yet very fulfilling.

Preparation Time: 10 minutes

Makes: 2 servings

Ingredient List:

- Chunk light tuna in water (4 oz.)
- Spicy brown mustard (1 teaspoon)
- Dijon mustard (2 teaspoons)
- Yellow mustard (2 teaspoons)
- Baby spinach (4 cups)
- Chopped carrots (1 cup)
- Chopped celery (1 cup)

Instructions:

Take a medium sized bowl and put chopped carrots and celery in it. Drain the water from the tuna and add the tuna to the carrots and celery.

Now add all the 3 kinds of mustards mentioned above. Mix the ingredients well.

When the ingredients are thoroughly mixed, put the baby spinach on a plate and top it with the salad mixture that you have just prepared. Enjoy your low cholesterol fish salad.

8) Garlic Basil Shrimp

If you are a shrimp lover like me, you would never want to eat anything else. This recipe would keep your cholesterol in check with just 53 mg of cholesterol. It is a versatile dish that you and your family members would fall in love with.

Preparation Time: 20 minutes

Makes: 4 servings

Ingredient List:

- 20 large shrimps
- Dry white wine (6 fl oz.)
- Grape tomatoes (6 oz.)
- 3 minced garlic cloves
- Salt (1 dash)
- Fresh ground pepper (1 dash)
- Olive oil (2 tablespoons)
- Fresh basil leaves (6 tablespoons)

zzzzzzzzzzzzzzzzzzzzzzzzzzzzzzzzzzzzzzzzz

Instructions:

Heat the olive oil in a large skillet over the medium-high heat. Make sure the oil is not too hot. Sauté the shrimps in oil, turning once. Cook them for 2 minutes.

When the shrimps have been cooked, transfer them to a bowl. Sauté the garlic and red pepper flakes in the remaining oil in the skillet for 30 seconds. Add wine and increase the heat.

Cook for 3 minutes. Stir in between. Add freshly chopped basil and tomatoes. Sprinkle salt and pepper. Return the shrimps to the skillet. Serve when the shrimps are thoroughly cooked.

9) Grilled Cilantro Salmon

You would especially enjoy this low calorie and low cholesterol recipe in summers because summer is for grilled salmon. This salmon recipe is just full of lots of delicious flavors.

Preparation Time: 45 minutes

Makes: 6 servings

Ingredient List:

- 4 salmon steaks
- 2 chopped garlic cloves
- Chopped cilantro leaves (1 bunch)
- Juice from one lime
- Honey (2 cups)
- Salt
- Pepper

zzzzzzzzzzzzzzzzzzzzzzzzzzzzzzzzzzzzzzzzzz

Instructions:

Over medium-low heat, stir together garlic, honey, lime juice and cilantro in a small saucepan. Cook for about 5 minutes until the honey can be stirred easily. Remove the mixture from heat and let it cool down. Season the salmon steaks with salt and pepper and place them on a baking sheet.

Pour the honey mixture over the salmon fish and put it in the refrigerator for 10 minutes. Meanwhile, preheat your outdoor grill on high heat. Oil the grill grate and place the fish steaks on the grill.

Take at least 5 minutes to cook each side of the fish. Check with a fork if the fish is cooked thoroughly. Enjoy this delicious grilled fish!

10) Parmesan Crusted Tilapia

It looks yummy, doesn't it? You can eat this yummy Tilapia without having to worry about your cholesterol level. This recipe only contains 47 mg of cholesterol.

Preparation Time: 25 minutes

Makes: 3 servings

Ingredient List:

- Tilapia (½ lb)
- Parmesan cheese (1/3 cup)
- Lime juice of 1 medium lime
- Olive oil (2 tablespoons)
- Salt
- Pepper

zzzzzzzzzzzzzzzzzzzzzzzzzzzzzzzzzzzzzzzzz

Instructions:

First of all, preheat your oven to 450 °F. Then wash the fish clean and tap it with a paper towel to dry it. Season it with salt and pepper. Then bake the fish for 5 minutes. Meanwhile, mix lime juice and olive oil together.

Pour this mixture over the fish and garnish with some parmesan cheese. Broil the fish for 2 minutes until you can see the top of the fish turning brown. Serve this yummy dish warm.

Chapter III: Low Cholesterol Beverages and Snacks

zzzzzzzzzzzzzzzzzzzzzzzzzzzzzzzzzzzzzzzzzzzz

11) Summer Breeze

You can see by the name of this beverage that it is a summer recipe. If you want to beat the bristling summer heat, you would want this drink. It has no cholesterol and just the look of it would make your mouth watery!

Preparation Time: 5 minutes

Makes: 3 servings

Ingredient List:

- Diced watermelon (5 cups)
- Blueberries (1.5 cups)
- 3 fresh basil leaves (1.5g)
- Lime (33.5g)
- Cayenne Pepper (2 pinches)

zzzzzzzzzzzzzzzzzzzzzzzzzzzzzzzzzzzzzzzzzzz

Instructions:

Take your juicer and put all the ingredients in it.

Blend until you get a smooth juicy fluid. Stir before you drink up!

12) Baked Sweet Potato Fries

Are you a fan of fries? Well, who isn't? These fries are better than the fries you eat in fast food restaurants. These have 0 mg of cholesterol and are a perfect substitute for salty and high-fat fries that you often crave. This recipe is quick and really simple.

Preparation Time: 40 minutes

Makes: 1 serving

Ingredient List:

- 1 sweet potato (5 inches long)
- Olive oil (1 tablespoon)
- Seasoned salt (¼ teaspoons)
- Paprika (1 teaspoon)
- Cumin (1 teaspoon)
- Cayenne pepper (1 dash)

zzzzzzzzzzzzzzzzzzzzzzzzzzzzzzzzzzzzzzzzzzz

Instructions:

Before you start working with the ingredients, set your oven to 400° F. Cut the sweet potato in long finger-like chips.

Now, take a big bowl and mix all the ingredients and sweet potato chips that you have cut. Mix the ingredients until the potatoes are covered with the spices evenly. Oil the baking sheet and spread the potato chips on the sheet in a single layer.

Bake them for 30 minutes. Eat with your favorite sauce or ketchup!

13) Peach Medley

Doesn't it look delicious? This yummy peach medley is rich in vitamin A, vitamin C, potassium, iron, dietary fibers and other nutrients. It has no cholesterol and is best to quench your thirst during hot summer days.

Preparation Time: 5 minutes

Makes: 4 servings

Ingredient List:

- 2 large peaches (350 g)
- 2 large apples (446g)
- 1 peeled lemon (42g)
- 1o medium carrots (610g)
- 1 large orange (184g)
- Ice

zzzzzzzzzzzzzzzzzzzzzzzzzzzzzzzzzzzzzzzzzzzz

Instructions:

To make this yummy peach medley, blend all the ingredients mentioned above in a juicer until you get a pulpy fluid.

Put ice in 4 glasses and pour the juice into the glasses. Stir before serving.

14) Crunchy Onion Rings

Looks good, eh? This recipe contains 0% cholesterol and it is the perfect snack that you can quickly make and enjoy in between your meals. I love crunchy onion rings because they are quick to make and they are extra delicious.

Preparation Time: 30 minutes

Makes: 1 serving

Ingredient List:

- 1 large onion
- Fiber One cereal (½ cup)
- 1 large egg
- Cooking spray

zzzzzzzzzzzzzzzzzzzzzzzzzzzzzzzzzzzzzzzz

Instructions:

First, set your oven to a temperature of 375° F. Meanwhile, remove the edges and the outer layer of the onion.

Make rings from the onion by cutting the onion into half-inch wide slices. Separate the layers to get onion rings. Set them aside. Grind the cereal in a food blender or processor until you get a breadcrumbs-like texture. Collect the crumbs into a dish. Take a small bowl and crack an egg into it. Beat the egg.

Now, one by one, dip each onion ring in the egg and then coat with the cereal crumbs. Spray an oven-safe baking dish with cooking spray and place the onion rings covered with cereal crumbs on it. Put the baking sheet in the oven for 25 minutes. Flip the onion rings halfway through the cooking. Your quick and yummy snack is ready. Enjoy!

15) Viva Forever!

You would find this low cholesterol beverage absolutely yummy and full of flavors. It's perfect for the start of the day. I love it, you would too!

Preparation Time: 5 minutes

Makes: 2 servings

Ingredient List:

- 12 medium carrots (732g)
- Ginger Root (24g)
- Cilantro (34g)
- Lemon (14.5g)
- Coconut Water (½ cup)
- Cayenne Pepper (¼ teaspoons)
- Lime (16.75g)
- Salt (0.4g)
- Ice

zzzzzzzzzzzzzzzzzzzzzzzzzzzzzzzzzzzzzzzzzzz

Instructions:

To make this healthy drink, add all the ingredients given above in a juicer and blend them well.

Add ice to glasses and pour the juice on top. Stir, sip and enjoy!

Chapter IV: Low Cholesterol Vegetarian Recipes

zzzzzzzzzzzzzzzzzzzzzzzzzzzzzzzzzzzzzzzzzz

16) Roasted Harvest Vegetables

Looks amazing, right? I love how this recipe is so colorful and so nutritious. This recipe will help you keep your cholesterol level to the lowest point. It contains 0 mg of cholesterol. With so many vegetables, this recipe is full of colorful and yummy flavors.

Preparation Time: 50 minutes

Makes: 9 servings

Ingredient List:

- Fresh cauliflowers (1 cup)
- Sliced medium yellow summer squash (1 cup)
- 2 quartered small onions
- 1 halved and sliced medium zucchini
- 8 quartered small red potatoes
- Fresh baby carrots (½ lb)
- Crushed dried rosemary (1 ½ teaspoons)
- Flowerets broccoli (1 cup)
- Pepper (¼ teaspoons)
- Salt (¼ teaspoons)
- Garlic powder (1 tablespoon)
- Dried thyme (½ teaspoons)
- Olive oil (¼ cup)

zzzzzzzzzzzzzzzzzzzzzzzzzzzzzzzzzzzzzzzzzz

Instructions:

Take a large bowl and put all the vegetables in it. Mix the rest of the spices and ingredients in a small bowl and sprinkle the mixture over the vegetables. Toss the vegetables to coat all the vegetables evenly.

Now, take two separate baking pans and grease them with olive oil. Transfer these vegetables to the baking pans. Don't cover the pans and let the vegetables bake for 30 minutes at 400° F. Stir the vegetables in between.

17) French Ratatouille

Yummm... This recipe would give you a watery mouth. It contains zero cholesterol and it's extremely delicious. You can enjoy this delicious vegetable mixture with pasta or eat it rolled inside an omelet too.

Preparation Time: 1 hour and 25 minutes

Makes: 15 servings

Ingredient List:

- Diced tomatoes (7 cups)
- 2 medium summer squash
- 3 large bell peppers
- 15 basil leaves
- 2 large zucchinis
- 2 peeled eggplants
- 2 large yellow onions
- Tomato paste (4 oz.)
- Olive oil (2 tablespoons)
- 4 garlic cloves

zzzzzzzzzzzzzzzzzzzzzzzzzzzzzzzzzzzzzzzzzzzz

Instructions:

Heat olive oil in a large skillet over medium-high heat. Then add thinly sliced onions in the skillet and cook them for 4 minutes until the onions start to soften up. Add diced bell peppers to the skillet and cook them along with the onions for another 4 minutes. In a large skillet, heat olive oil over the medium-high heat.

Now, dice the summer squash and zucchini just the way you diced the bell peppers. Add them to the skillet and cook for 5 minutes. Take the eggplant and if you like, you can keep the skin on it. Dice the eggplant and toss it into the skillet. Cook for 7 minutes.

Add diced garlic and stir to mix the vegetables well. Add tomato paste and diced tomatoes. Stir to mix. Season with salt and pepper according to your taste.

Let all the vegetables to simmer for 40 minutes until the vegetables are all soft and the mixture is thick enough. Now, make thin strips of basil. Remove from heat and stir the vegetables. Enjoy!

18) Balsamic and Olive Oil Roasted Brussels sprouts

This recipe is very tasty. If you are a vegetarian and you are bored eating vegetables cooked the same way, you would love these roasted Brussels sprouts that have no cholesterol.

Preparation Time: 30 minutes

Makes: 4 servings

Ingredient List:

- Brussels sprouts (1 lb.)
- Balsamic vinegar (2 tablespoons)
- Olive oil (1 tablespoon)
- Pepper
- Salt
- 1 garlic clove
- Cooking spray

zzzzzzzzzzzzzzzzzzzzzzzzzzzzzzzzzzzzzzzzzz

Instructions:

Set your oven to a temperature of 375° F. Then grease the baking dish with cooking spray. Trim the Brussels sprouts and cut each sprout in two equal pieces. Put the sprouts in the baking dish and flip with olive oil, 1 tablespoon of balsamic vinegar and garlic.

Now, roast the sprouts in the oven for 10 minutes. Open the oven, stir the sprouts and roast them for another 10 minutes. Collect the sprouts in a serving bowl and sprinkle 1 tablespoon of balsamic vinegar over them. Garnish with salt and pepper according to your taste. Enjoy!

19) Creamy Corn Casserole

This yummy and creamy casserole is perfect for vegetable lovers. It contains only 10 mg of cholesterol. This yummy casserole with fill your mouth with a divine creamy flavor that you will fall in love with.

Preparation Time: 55 minutes

Makes: 4 servings

Ingredient List:

- Sweet corn (1 cup)
- Reduced fat Velveeta cheese (1 oz.)
- Crushed saltines (1/3 cup)
- Egg noodles (1 cup)
- Pepper (¼ tablespoons)
- Salt (¼ tablespoons)
- Cream corn (1 cup)
- Fat-free margarine (1 tablespoon)
- Cooking spray.

zzzzzzzzzzzzzzzzzzzzzzzzzzzzzzzzzzzzzzzzzzzz

Instructions:

Except for the crackers and the margarine, mix all the ingredients in a big bowl. Now, spray a baking dish with cooking spray and pour the ingredients into the baking dish. Spread them evenly throughout the baking sheet.

Sprinkle cracker crumbs and margarine over the mixture. Put the baking pan inside the oven and bake the casserole for 45 minutes at 350 °F. Check with a fork if everything is cooked through. Serve and enjoy!

20) All-Vegetable Soup

Are you a vegetarian and a soup lover?? This delicious recipe is solely for you. With 0 mg of cholesterol, this recipe is totally nutritious and tasty at the same time.

Preparation Time: 50 minutes

Makes: 12 servings

Ingredient List:

- Vegetable broth (6 cups)
- Shredded cabbage (2 cups)
- Chopped fresh thyme (2 teaspoons)
- 2 diced small zucchini
- Chopped Swiss chard (2 cups)
- Chopped small florets broccoli (2 cups)
- 2 chopped medium carrots
- Small florets cauliflower (2 cups)
- 1 chopped medium onion
- 1 diced stalk medium celery
- Chopped fresh parsley (2 tablespoons)
- 1 diced medium red bell pepper
- Lemon juice (½ fl oz.)
- Black pepper (¼ teaspoons)
- Table salt (½ teaspoons)
- 2 cloves garlic

zzzzzzzzzzzzzzzzzzzzzzzzzzzzzzzzzzzzzzzzzzz

Instructions:

Take a large soup pot and put all the vegetables, garlic, thyme and vegetable broth in it. Cover the pot and bring to boil over high heat. After the broth starts boiling, lower the heat, cover it and let it simmer for 10 minutes. After that, add parsley and stir. Sprinkle lemon juice if you like. Add salt and pepper according to your taste.

If you want your soup to be thick, you can puree it by blending all the vegetables in the soup. For that, use an immersion blender and puree the soup.

Chapter V: Low Cholesterol Desserts

zzzzzzzzzzzzzzzzzzzzzzzzzzzzzzzzzzzzzzzzzz

21) Mango Raspberry Sorbet

This absolutely yummy dessert is perfect for you if you love desserts and want to keep your cholesterol in check. This dessert contains 0 mg of cholesterol.

Preparation Time: 10 minutes

Makes: 1 serving

Ingredient List:

- Frozen mango (half a cup)
- Frozen raspberries (half a cup)
- Orange juice (half a cup)
- Mint sprig

zzzzzzzzzzzzzzzzzzzzzzzzzzzzzzzzzzzzzzzzzzz

Instructions:

In a blender, put all the ingredients mentioned above.

Blend the ingredients on high speed. Let the mixture blend until you get a smooth texture.

Spoon the sorbet into a cup and garnish with a mint sprig. Enjoy!

22) Chocolate Chip Oatmeal Cookies

I am a chocolate lover and these chocolate cookies are my love. I make these to my kids every other day. They love it. You would love it too. These cookies have only 5 mg of cholesterol.

Preparation Time: 1 hour and 13 minutes

Makes: 40 servings

Ingredient List:

- Cocoa powder (3 tablespoons)
- Oats (1 /4 cups)
- Chocolate chips (6 oz.)
- Brown sugar (½ cup)
- Unsifted confectioner's sugar (3/4 cup)
- 1 large egg
- Whole wheat flour (½ cup)
- Unsweetened applesauce (¼ cup)
- Baking soda (½ teaspoons)
- Baking powder (1 teaspoon)
- Cinnamon (½ teaspoons)
- Salt (½ teaspoons)
- Vanilla (1 teaspoon)
- Canola oil (¼ cup)
- All-purpose flour (½ cup)
- Cooking spray

ZZZZZZZZZZZZZZZZZZZZZZZZZZZZZZZZZZZZZZZZZZZ

Instructions:

Set your oven to heat to 350°F. Take out your baking sheets and coat them with cooking spray or you can also line them with parchment paper. Now, take a small bowl and add cocoa powder, all-purpose flour, baking powder, baking soda, whole-wheat flour, cinnamon and salt. Mix all the ingredients until they are well combined. Set this bowl aside and take another bowl, this time a large one and add oil, confectioners' sugar, brown sugar, vanilla, egg and applesauce to it.

Add this mixture to the flour mixture and mix both mixtures well until they are well-combined. Add chocolate chips and oats. Stir well. Take spoonful of this mixture and place them on the baking sheet that you have prepared. Leave 2 inches of space between each cookie.

Put the cookies in the preheated oven for 12 minutes until they are lightly brown. Make sure you don't over bake the cookies. Remove the cookies from the oven and let them cool down. Serve these cookies with tea or milk and enjoy!

23) Pumpkin Mousse

This recipe is absolutely delicious and is low in calories and fat. It contains only 2 mg of cholesterol.

Preparation Time: 1 hour and 15 minutes

Makes: 6 servings

Ingredient List:

- Pumpkin (1 cup)
- Fat-free evaporated milk (2/3 cup)
- Vanilla pudding and pie filling (1 package)
- Ground cinnamon (¼ teaspoons)
- Low fat frozen whipped topping (1 ½ cups)

zzzzzzzzzzzzzzzzzzzzzzzzzzzzzzzzzzzzzzzzzzz

Instructions:

In a bowl, mix evaporated milk, pumpkin, pudding mix and cinnamon until they are well combined. Add whipped topping gently into the mixture.

Cover the bowl and refrigerate for an hour before you serve this yummy dessert.

24) Zesty Lemon Bars

This cute-looking recipe tastes like a blessing. It is low in calories and has only 17 mg of cholesterol.

Preparation Time: 1 hour and 5 minutes

Makes: 16 servings

Ingredient List:

- 1 large lemon
- Baking powder (0.12 teaspoons)
- Light butter (2 oz.)
- 1 large egg
- 1 large egg white
- Salt (0.12 teaspoons)
- All-purpose flour (9 ½ oz.)
- Granulated sugar (3/4 cup)
- Confectioners' sugar (1 teaspoon)
- Cooking spray

zzzzzzzzzzzzzzzzzzzzzzzzzzzzzzzzzzzzzzzzzzzz

Instructions:

Spray an 8x8 baking pan with cooking spray. Heat your oven to 350 °F. In a bowl, mix ¼ cup of sugar, salt and 1 cup of flour until well combined. Add butter to the mixture and mix until crumbly dough is formed. Spread this dough evenly on the bottom of the prepared baking pan. Bake this dough until it's lightly golden. This would take 12 minutes.

Then, completely let it cool down. In a bowl, add an egg, an egg white and the remaining half cup of sugar. Whisk it well until it is combined. Add lemon juice and zest to the egg mixture. Add 3 tablespoons of flour and baking powder in the mixture. Stir thoroughly. Pour this liquid over the cool crust. Bake it for 25 minutes until the edges turn brown.

Collect from the oven and cool it down completely. Sprinkle powdered sugar on it. Cut into 16 square slices.

25) Strawberry Fluff

Looks beautiful, doesn't it? Being a strawberry fan, this one is my personal favorite with only 0 mg of cholesterol.

Preparation Time: 35 minutes

Makes: 12 servings

Ingredient List:

- Diced strawberries (4 cups)
- Sugar-free strawberry gelatin (1 tablespoon)
- Fat-free vanilla pudding (0.8 oz.)
- Fat-free tapioca (3 oz.)
- Water (2 ½ cups)
- Low-fat cool whip (8 oz.)

zzzzzzzzzzzzzzzzzzzzzzzzzzzzzzzzzzzzzzzzzz

Instructions:

In a saucepan, mix tapioca, vanilla pudding and gelatin. Add water and boil the mixture. Remove from heat and let it cool down.

Add the strawberries and cool whip to the gelatin mixture. Refrigerate before serving.

About the Author

A native of Albuquerque, New Mexico, Sophia Freeman found her calling in the culinary arts when she enrolled at the Sante Fe School of Cooking. Freeman decided to take a year after graduation and travel around Europe, sampling the cuisine from small bistros and family owned restaurants from Italy to Portugal. Her bubbly personality and inquisitive nature made her popular with the locals in the villages and when she finished her trip and came home, she had made friends for life in the places she had visited. She also came home with a deeper understanding of European cuisine.

Freeman went to work at one of Albuquerque's 5-star restaurants as a sous-chef and soon worked her way up to head chef. The restaurant began to feature Freeman's original dishes as specials on the menu and soon after, she began to write e-books with her recipes. Sophia's dishes mix local flavours with European inspiration making them irresistible to the diners in her restaurant and the online community.

Freeman's experience in Europe didn't just teach her new ways of cooking, but also unique methods of presentation. Using rich sauces, crisp vegetables and meat cooked to perfection, she creates a stunning display as well as a delectable dish. She has won many local awards for her cuisine and she continues to delight her diners with her culinary masterpieces.

* * * * ★ ★ ★ ★ * * *

Author's Afterthoughts

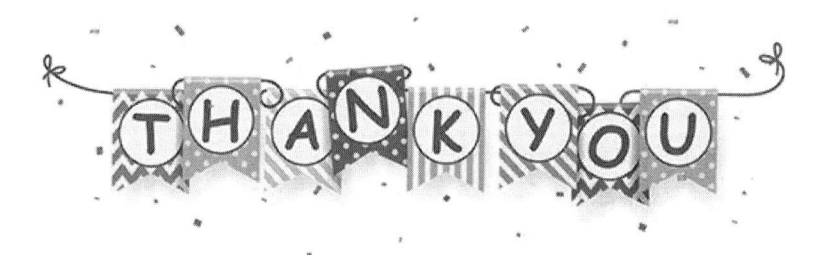

I want to convey my big thanks to all of my readers who have taken the time to read my book. Readers like you make my work so rewarding and I cherish each and every one of you.

Grateful cannot describe how I feel when I know that someone has chosen my work over all of the choices available online. I hope you enjoyed the book as much as I enjoyed writing it.

Feedback from my readers is how I grow and learn as a chef and an author. Please take the time to let me know your thoughts by leaving a review on Amazon so I and your fellow readers can learn from your experience.

My deepest thanks,

Sophia Freeman

Subscribe to the Newsletter!

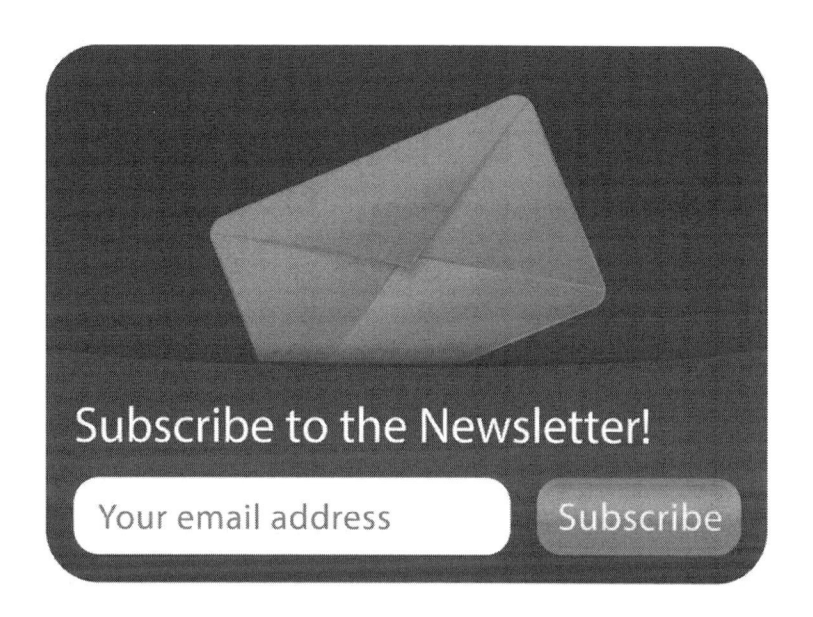

https://sophia.subscribemenow.com/

* * * * ★ ★ ★ ★ ★ * * * *

Printed in Great Britain
by Amazon